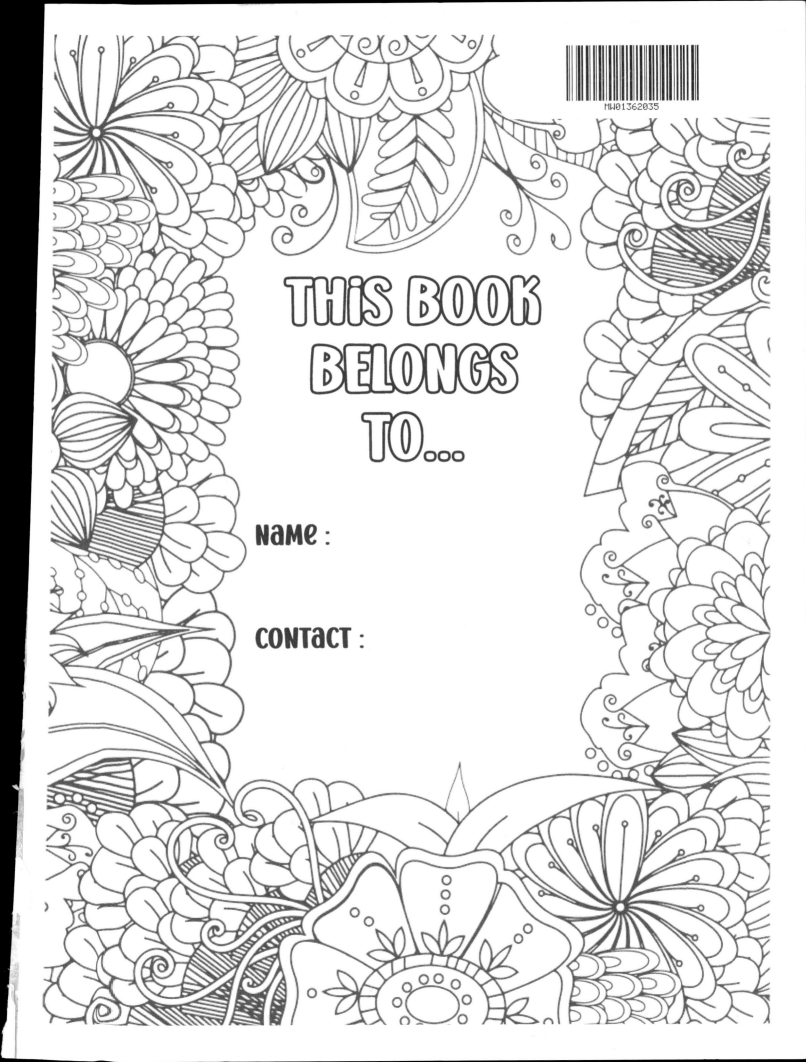

ISBN: 9798858649182

Copyright © 2023
ALL RIGHTS RESERVED.

No part of this publication may be reproduced or transmitted in any form or by any means telectronic or mechanical, including photocopying, recording or by any information storage and retrieval system, without written permission from publisher except in the case of brief quotations embodied in critical reviews and certain other non-commercial uses permitted by copyright law.

TEST THE COLORS

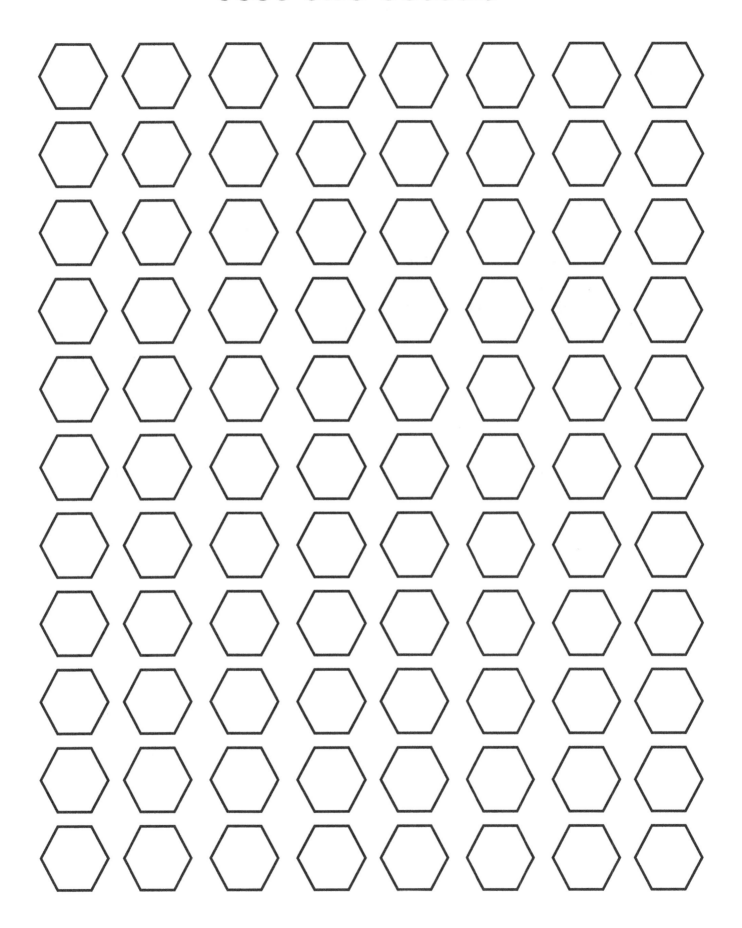

CARE FOR MOTHER NATURE

We understands our responsibility towards environment. We contribute for growing more trees and helps to improve nature. A small portion of your payment made towards this book, will also be used for this green cause.

SHARE WHAT YOU FEEL

Thank you for purchasing this book. Our team had dedicatedly worked out to make this book full of fun, excitement and creativity. We put in extensive efforts from hiring multiple high skilled illustrators and creative quote masters, to producing the book and bring it to you, ensuring a seamless and high-quality experience for you. If you are reading this, please take a moment and leave your honest review by going to your Amazon orders section. Your just one review will help us to further research and update the book and supports our business to grow. This will also help other buyers to know more about this book.

We are deeply grateful that you've take time and leave your valuable feedback.

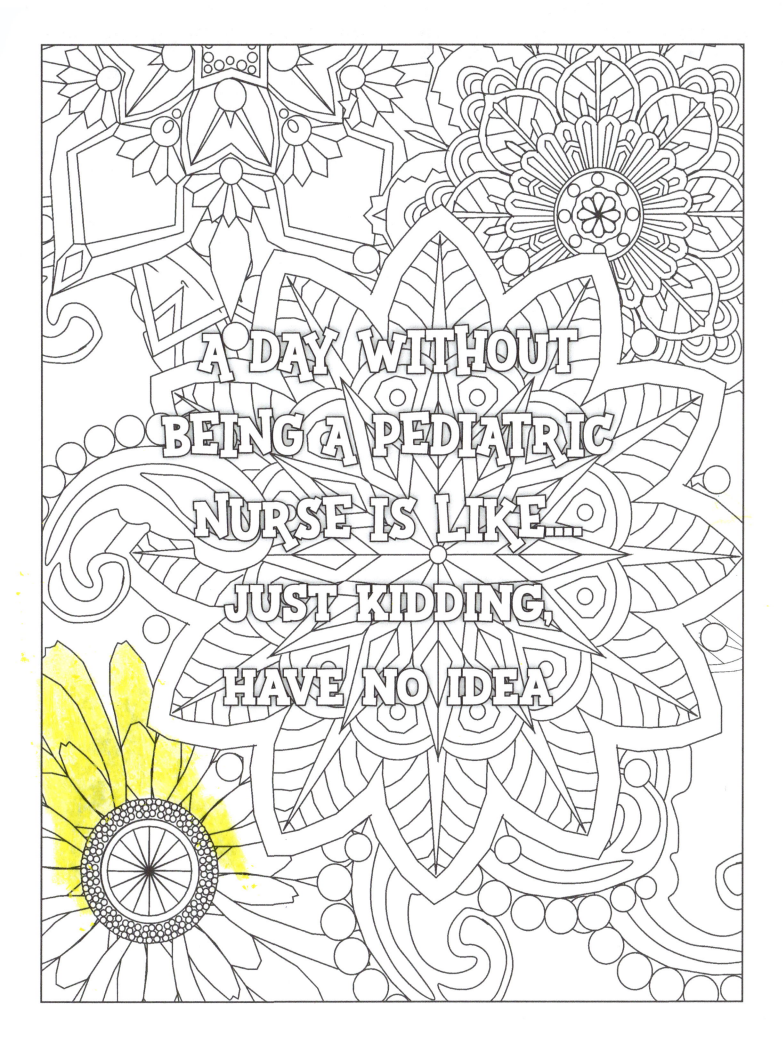

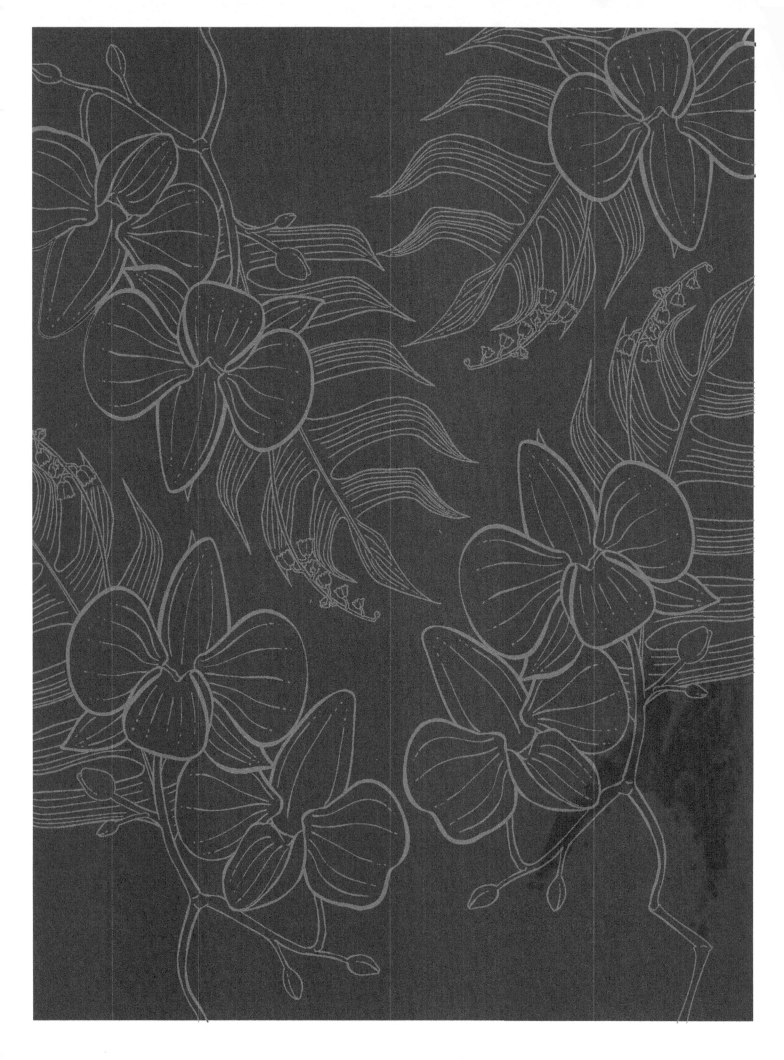

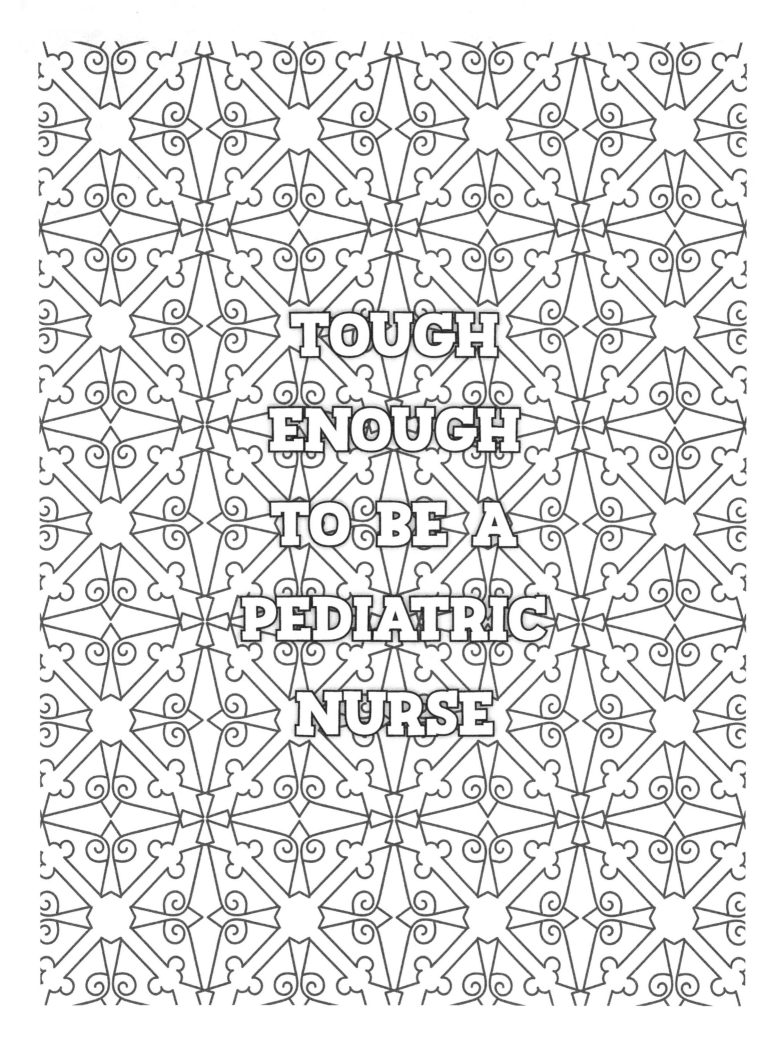

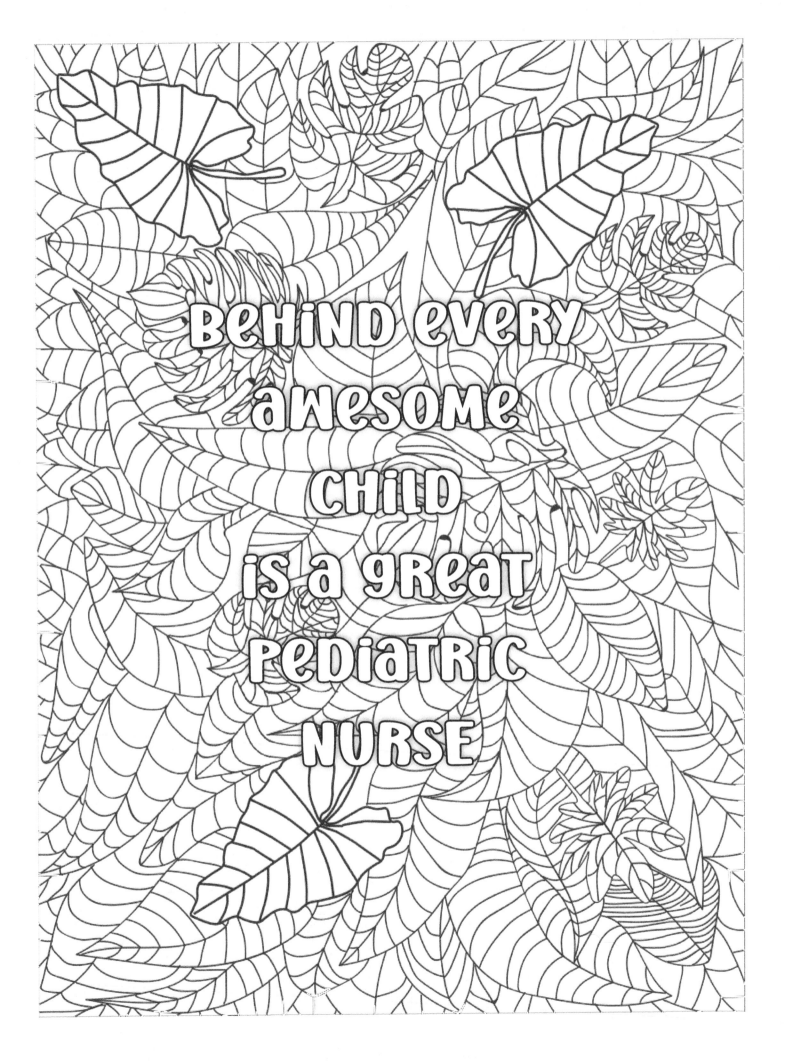

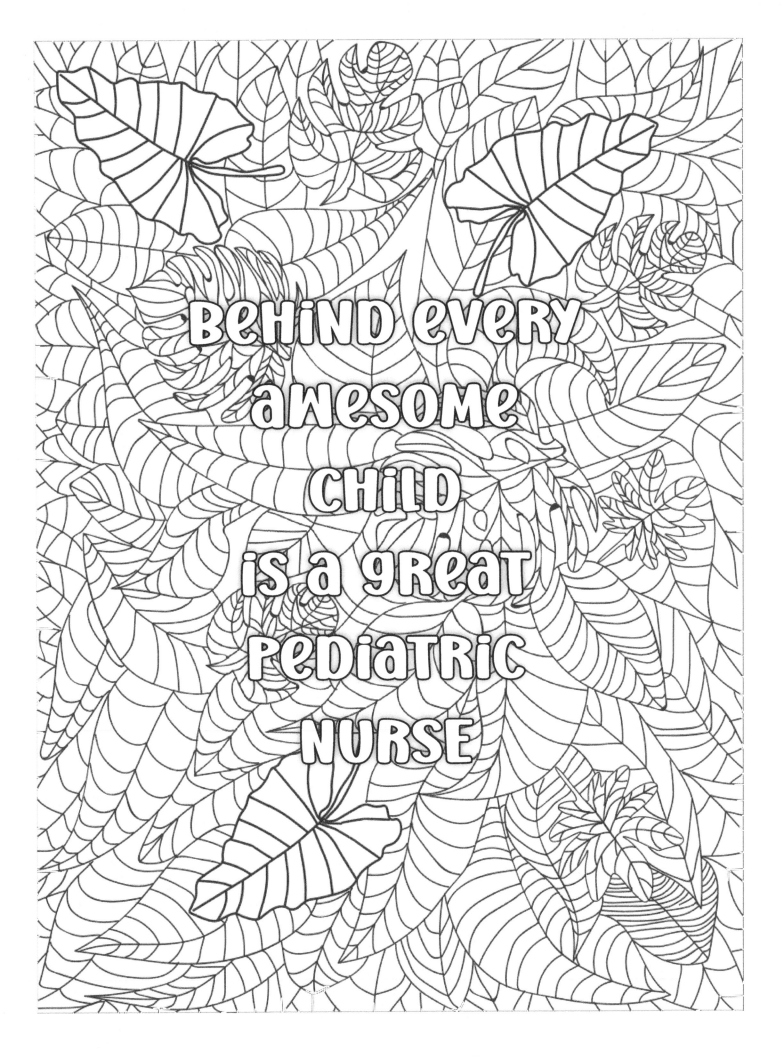

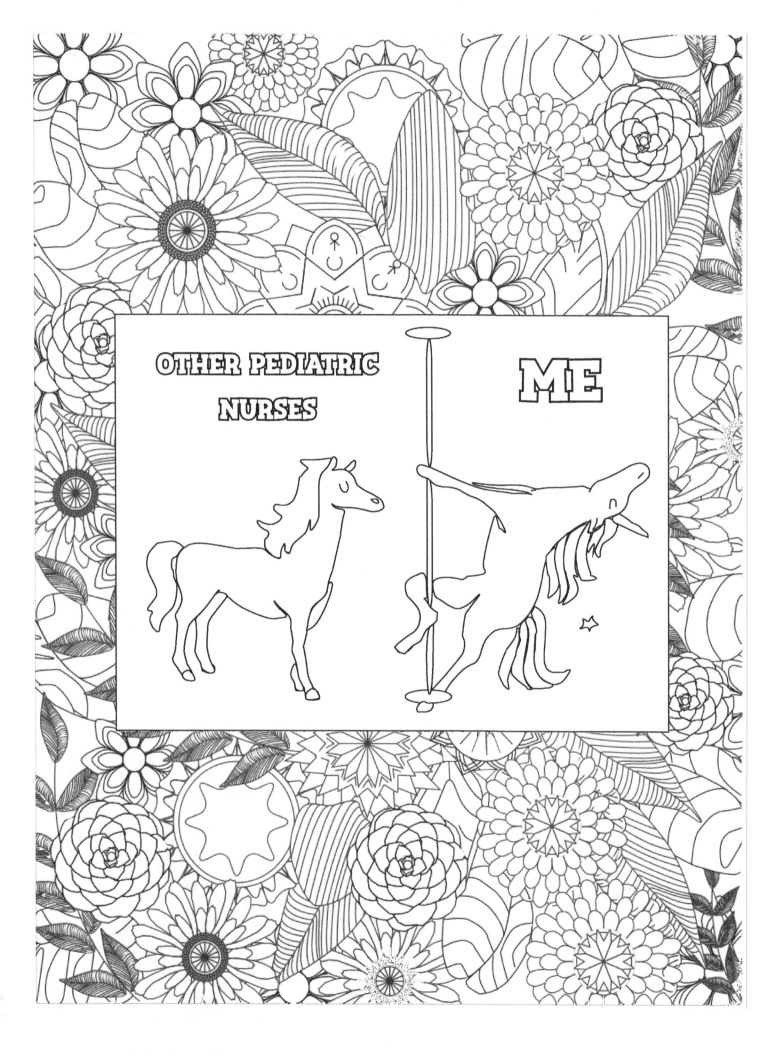

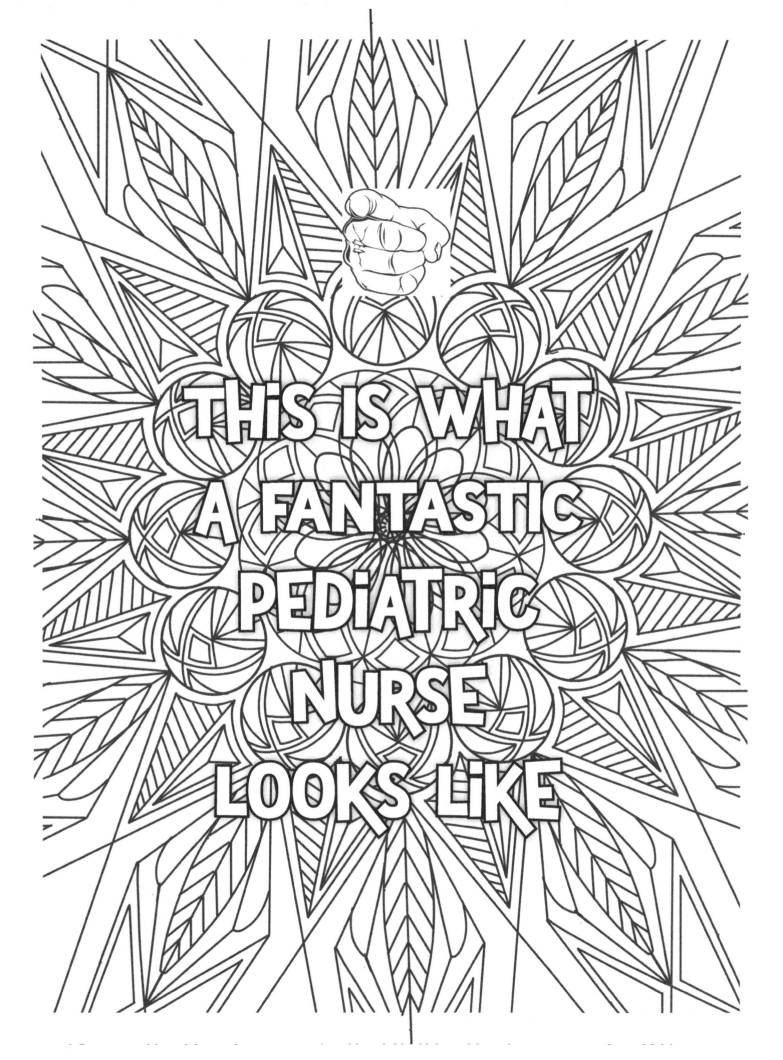

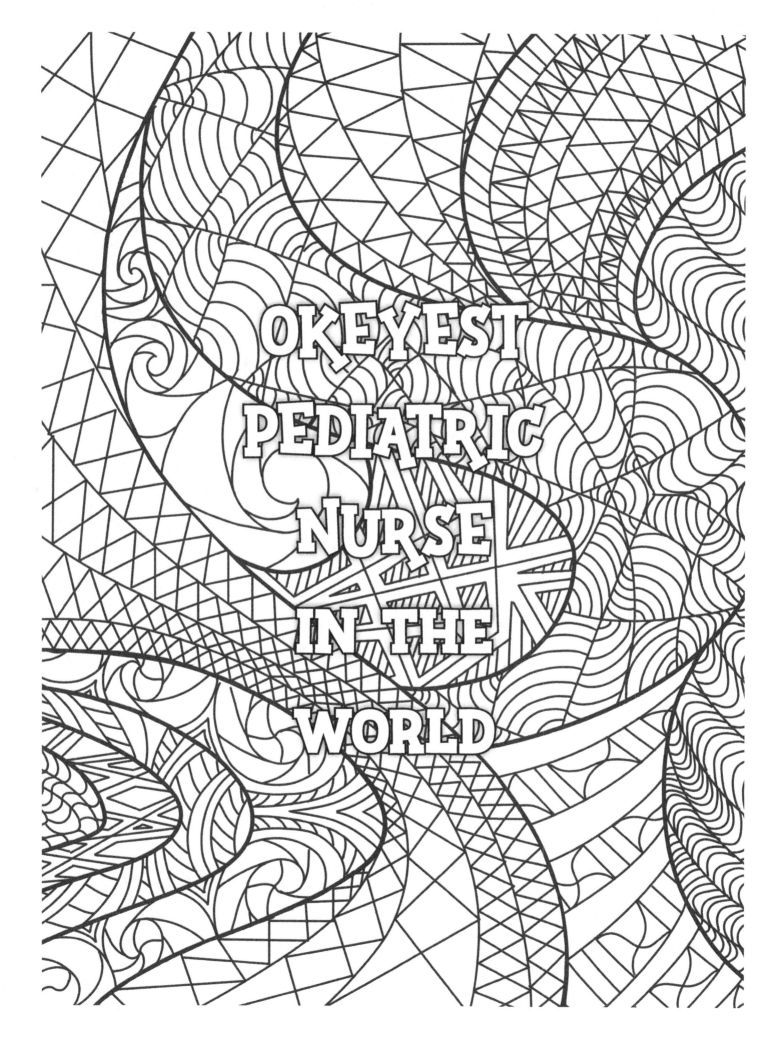

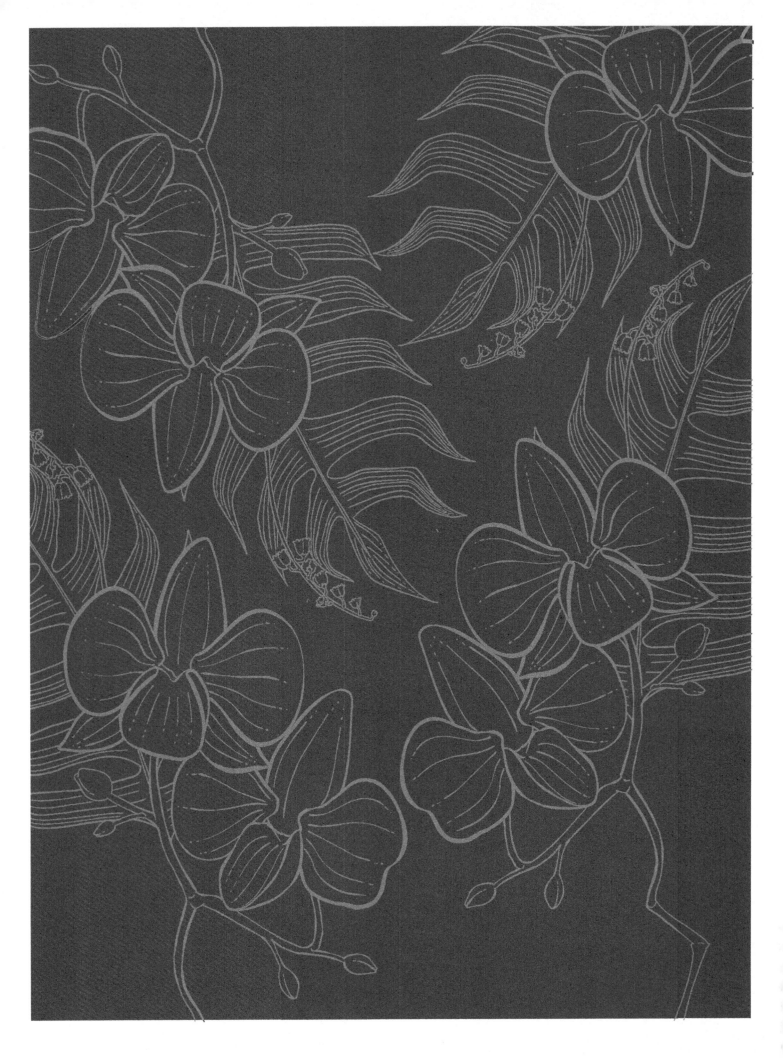

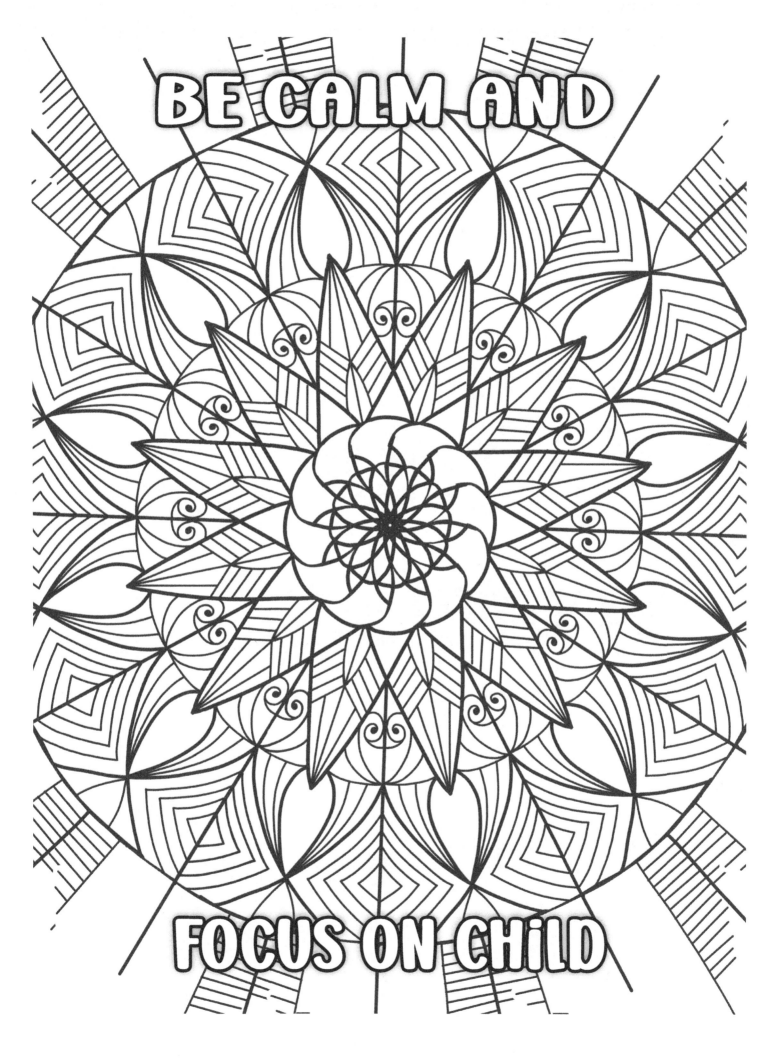

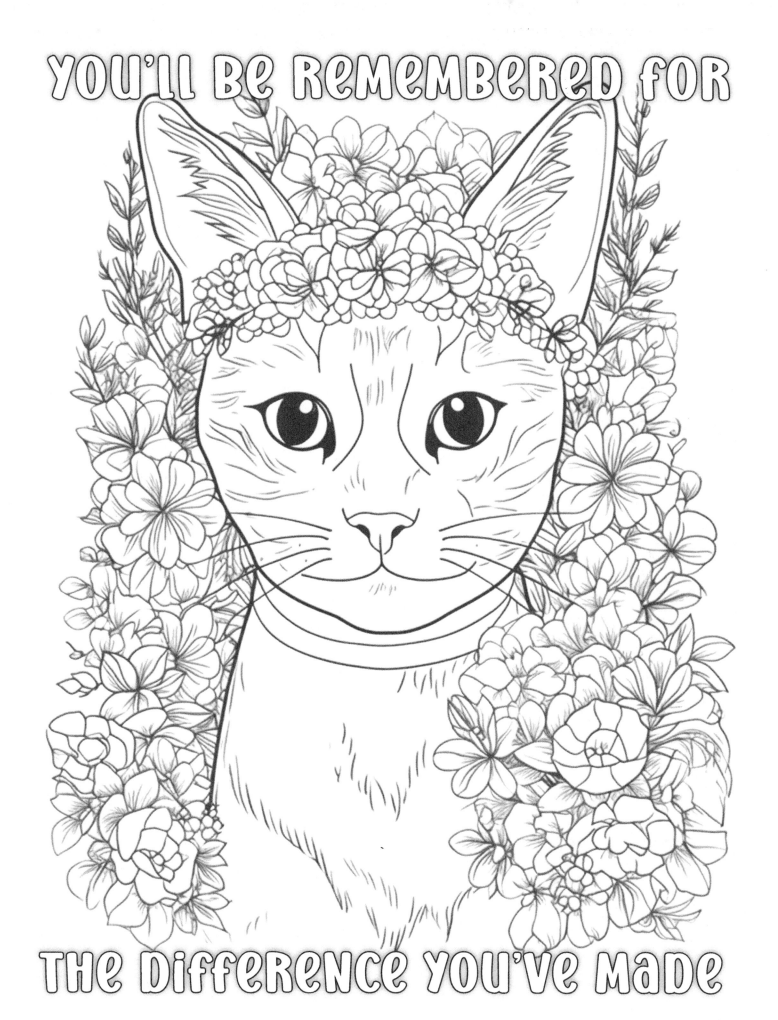

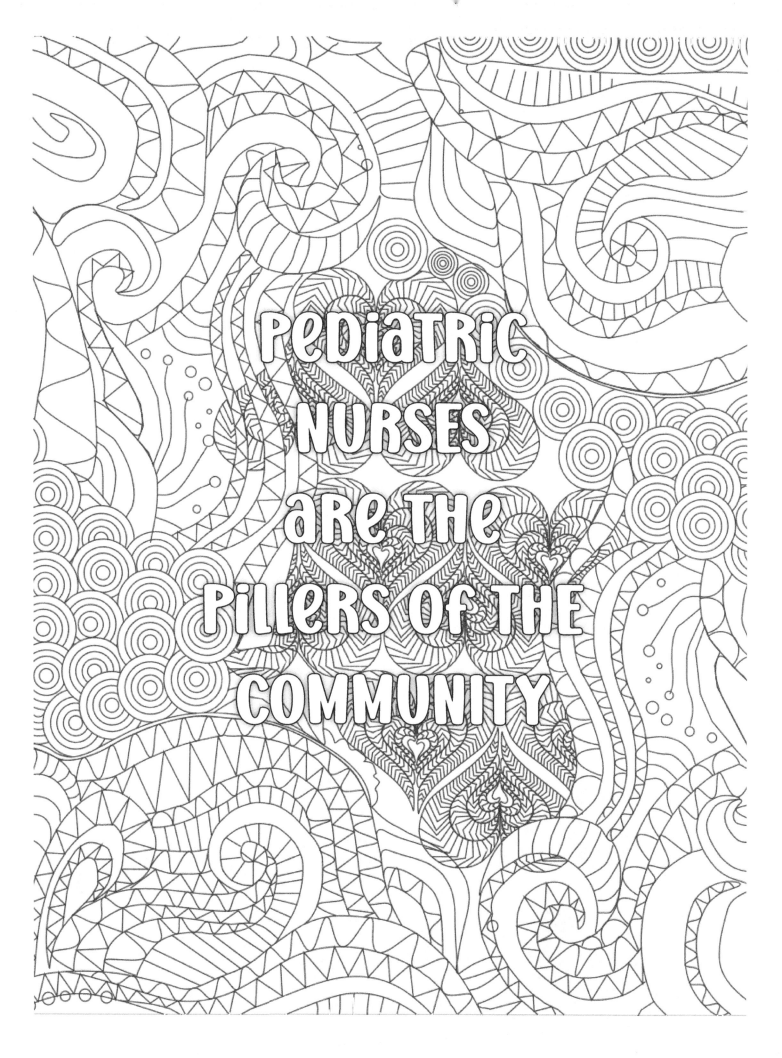

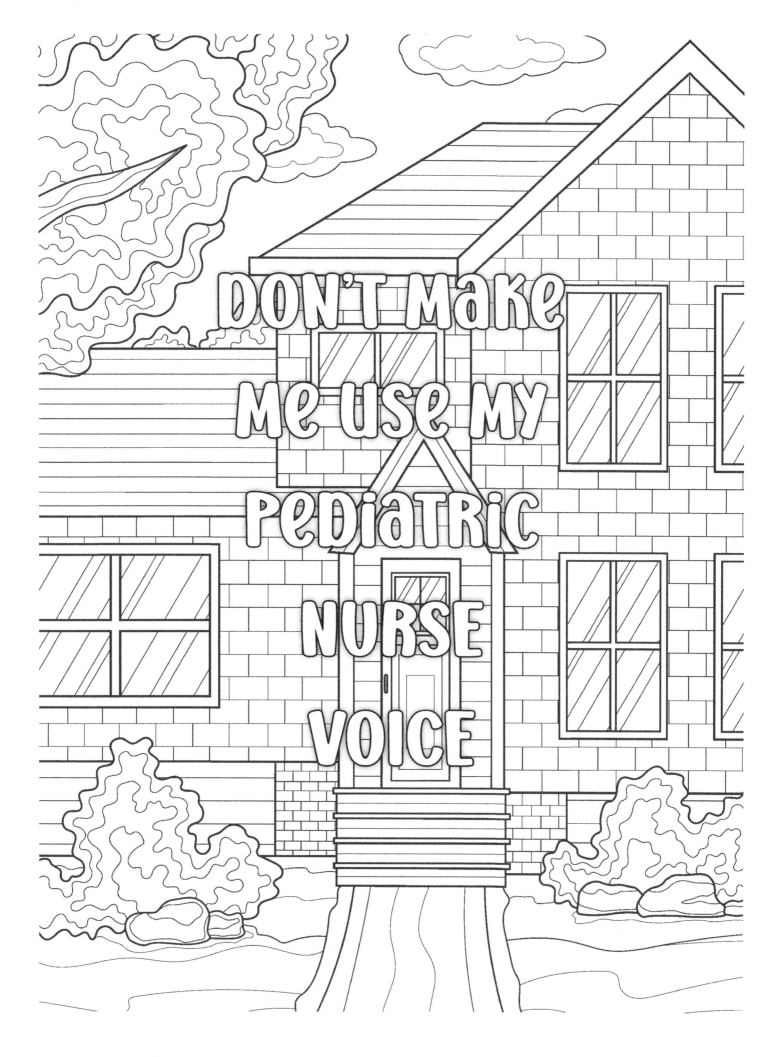

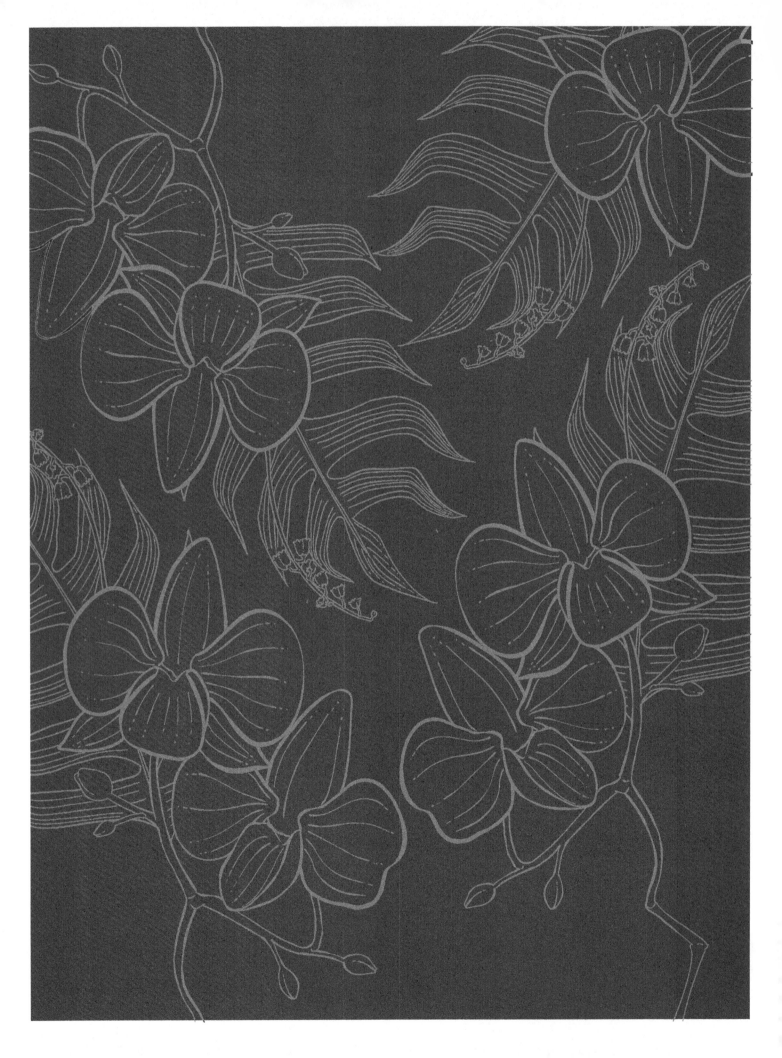

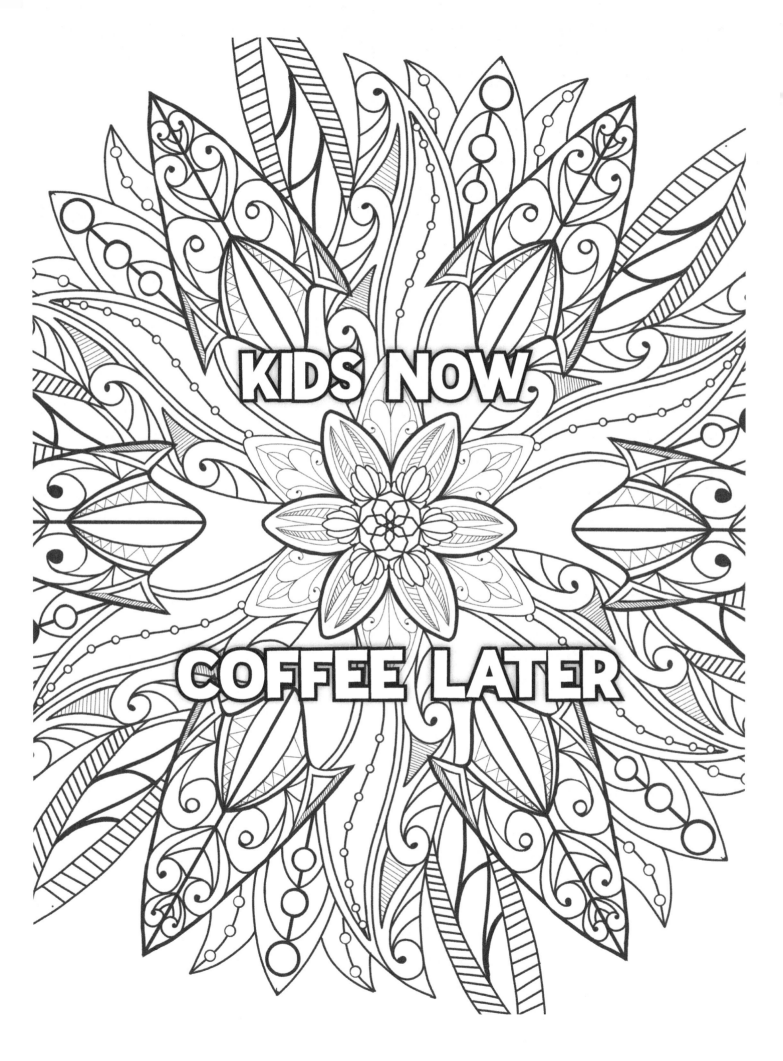

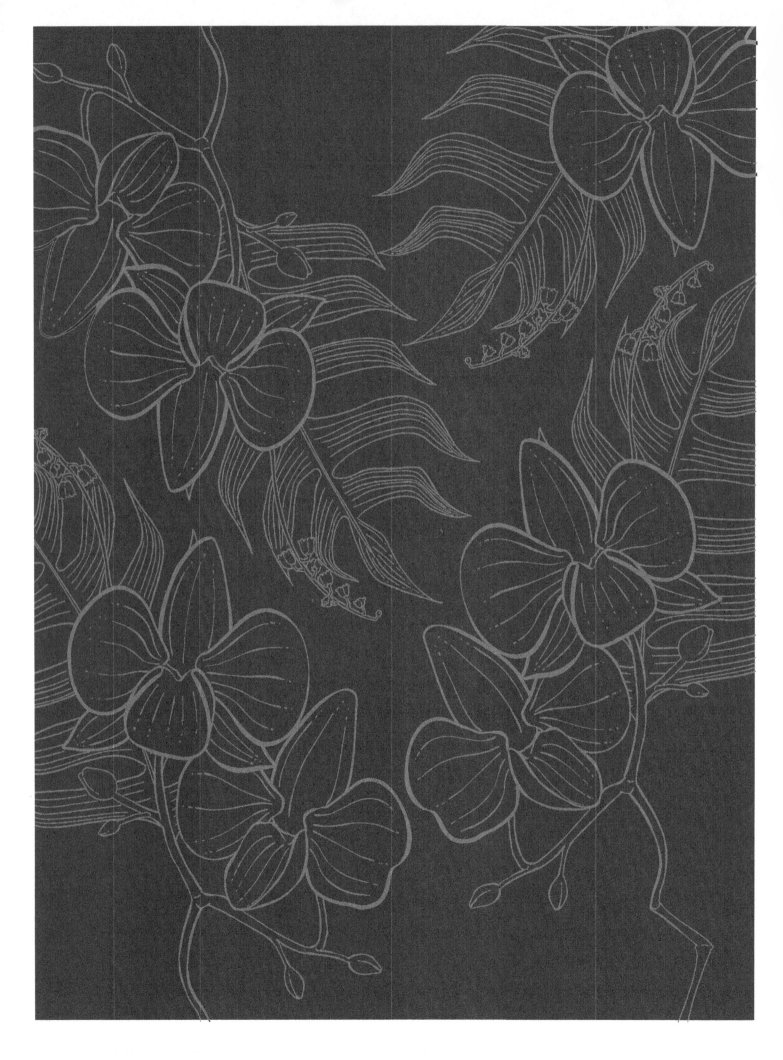

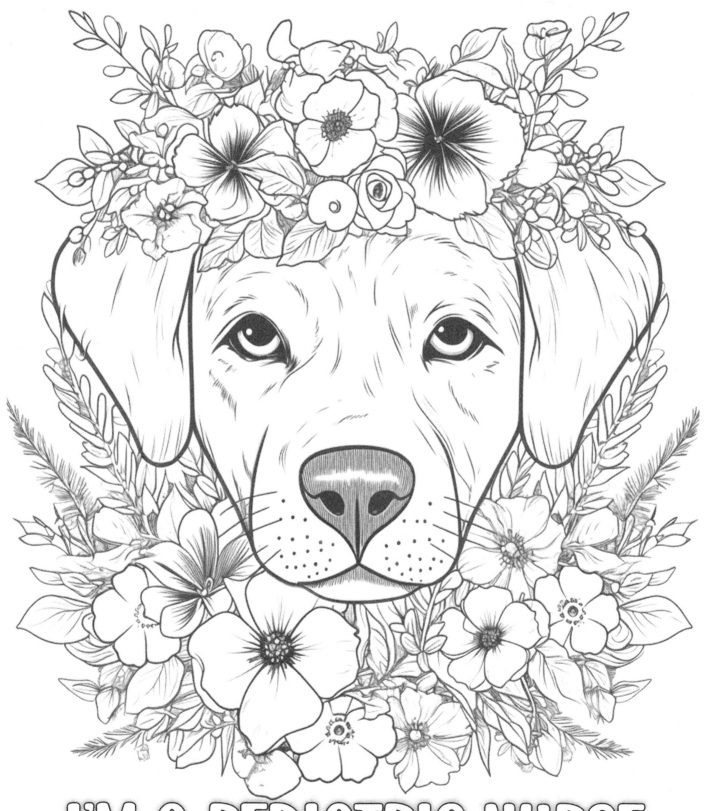

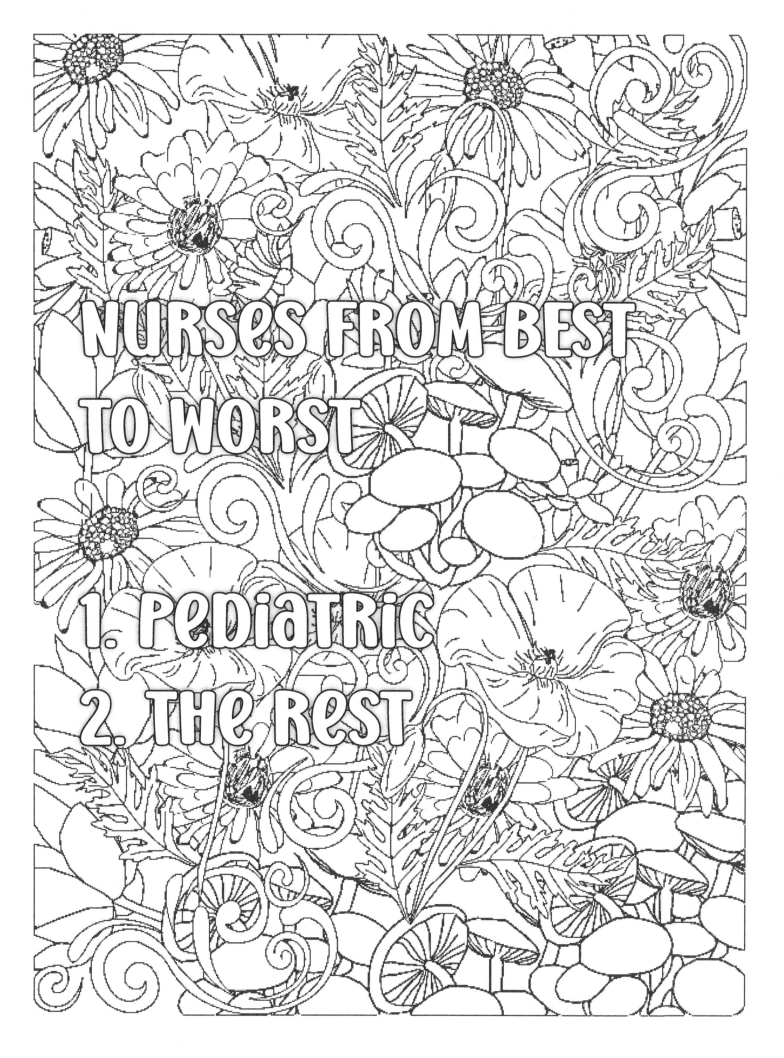

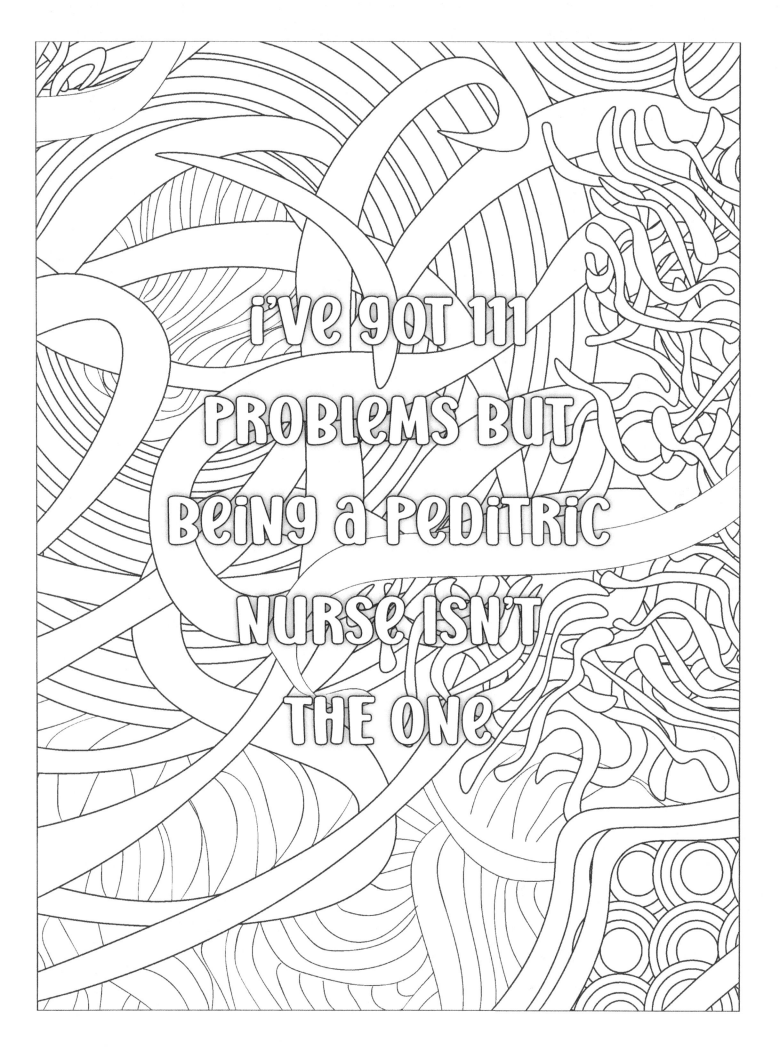

BEING A PEDIATRIC NURSE

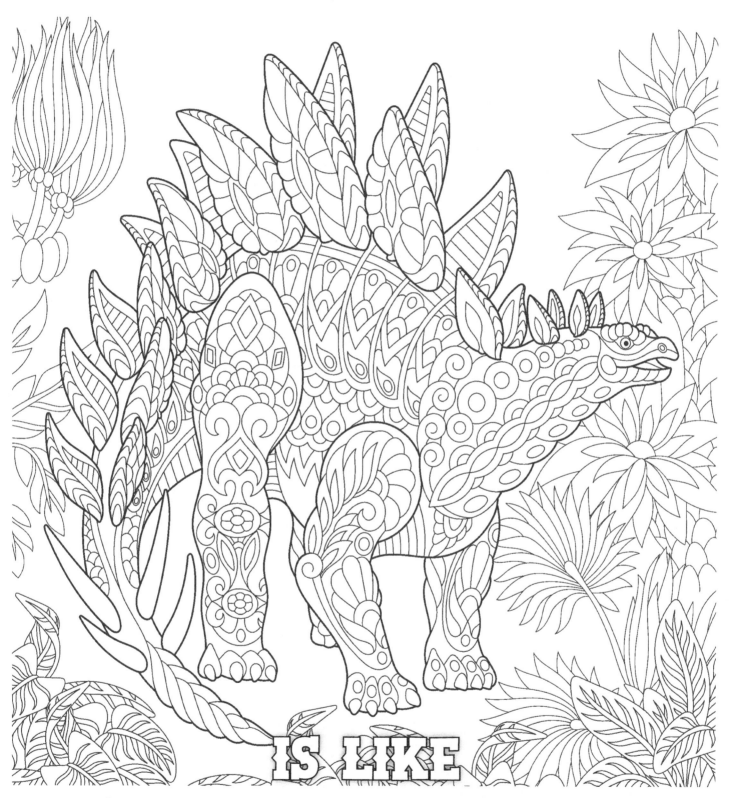

IS LIKE
WALKING IN THE PARK

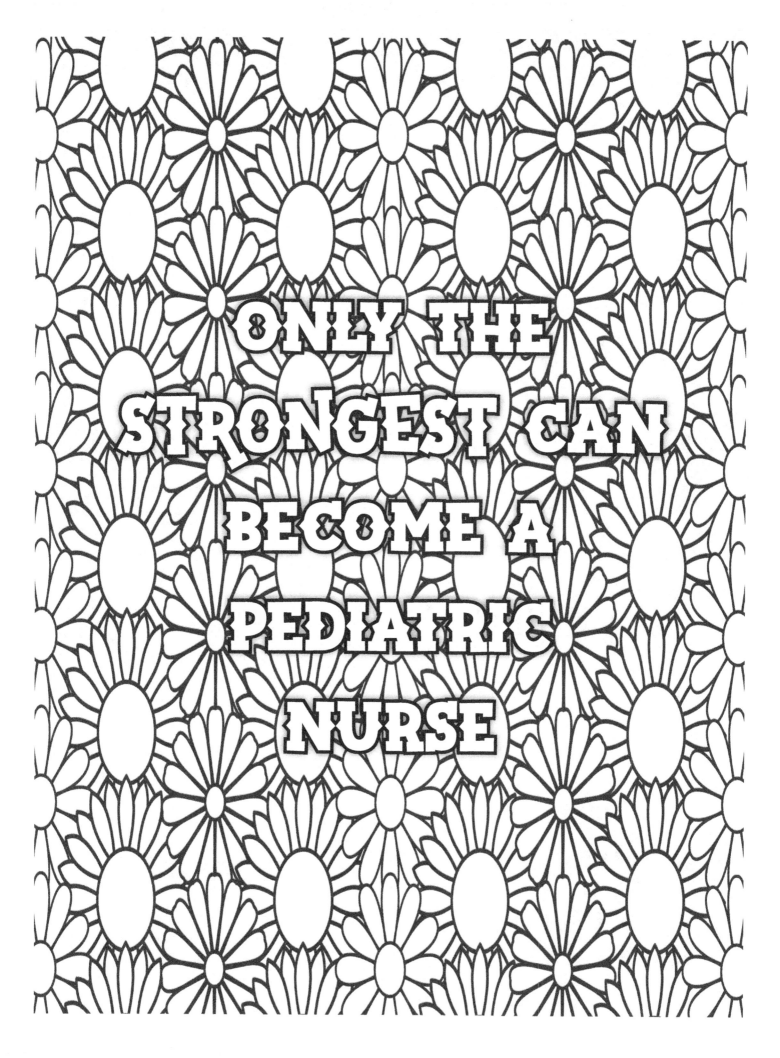

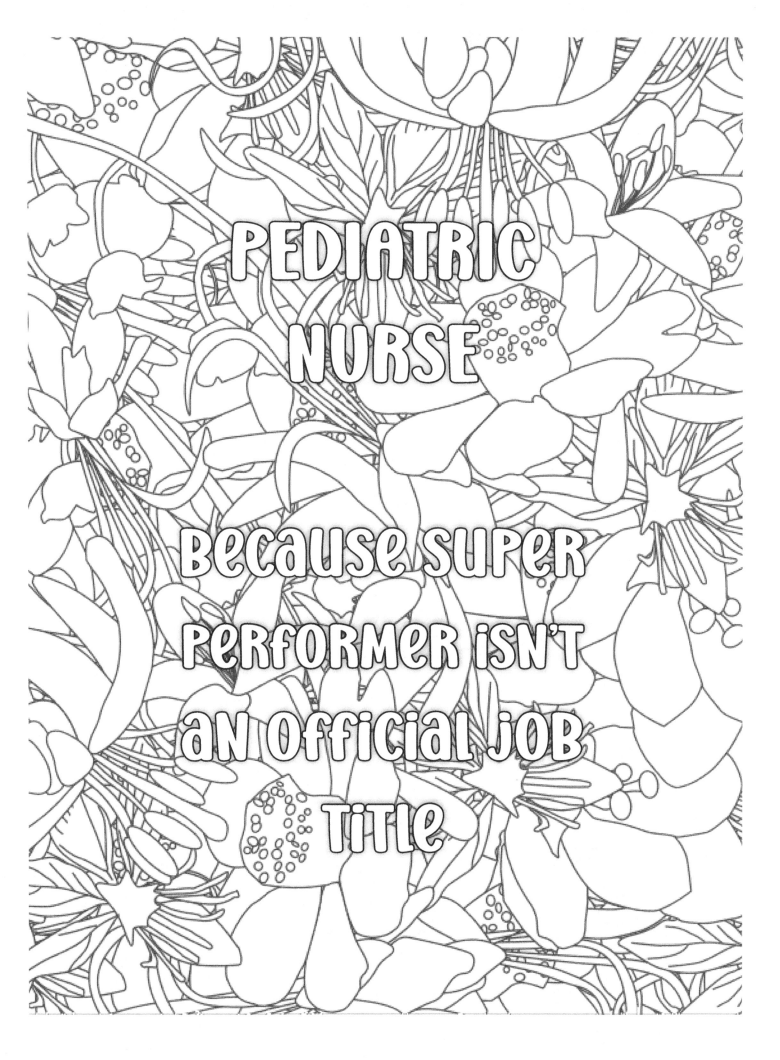

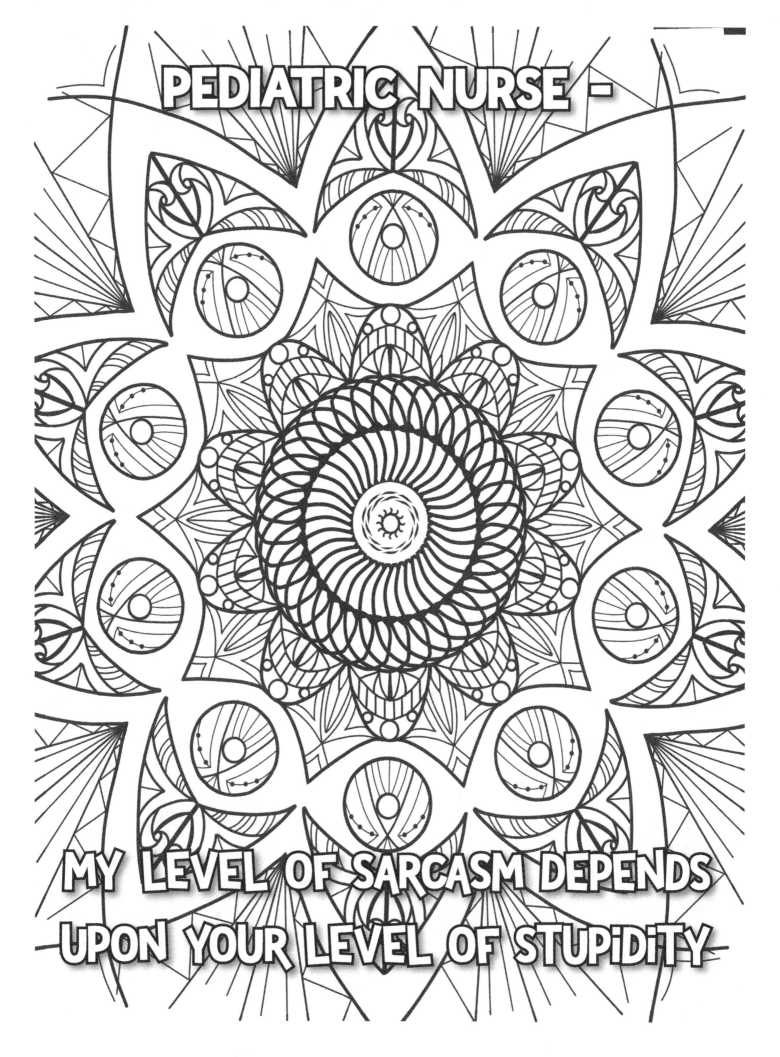

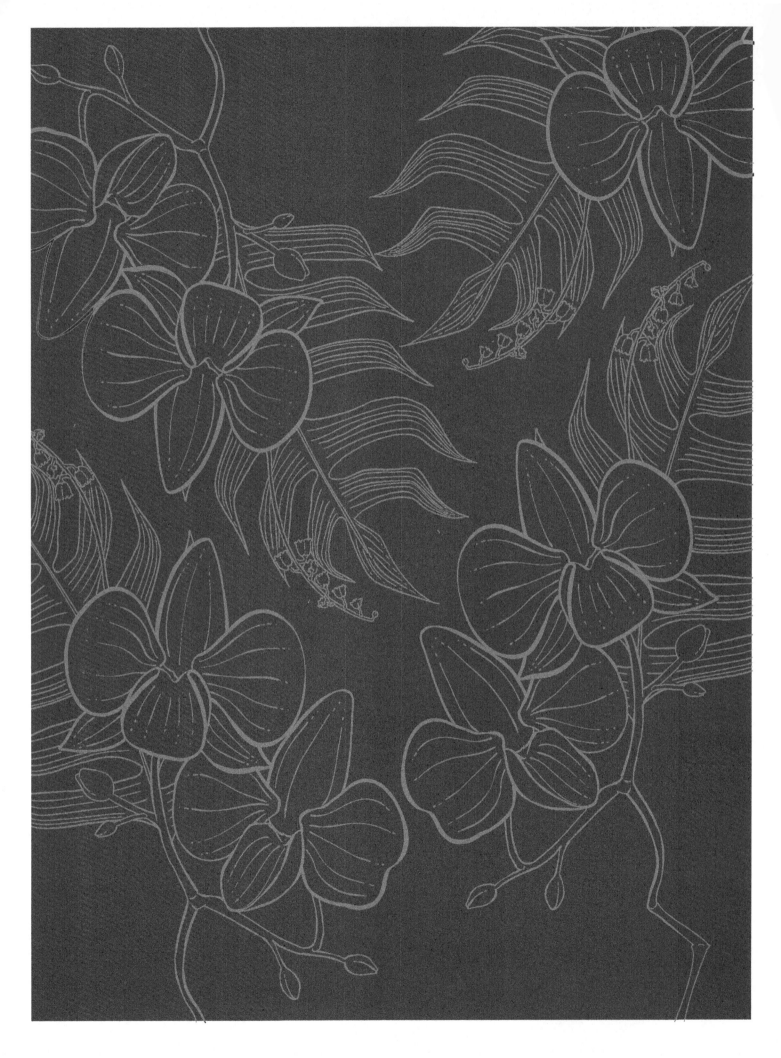

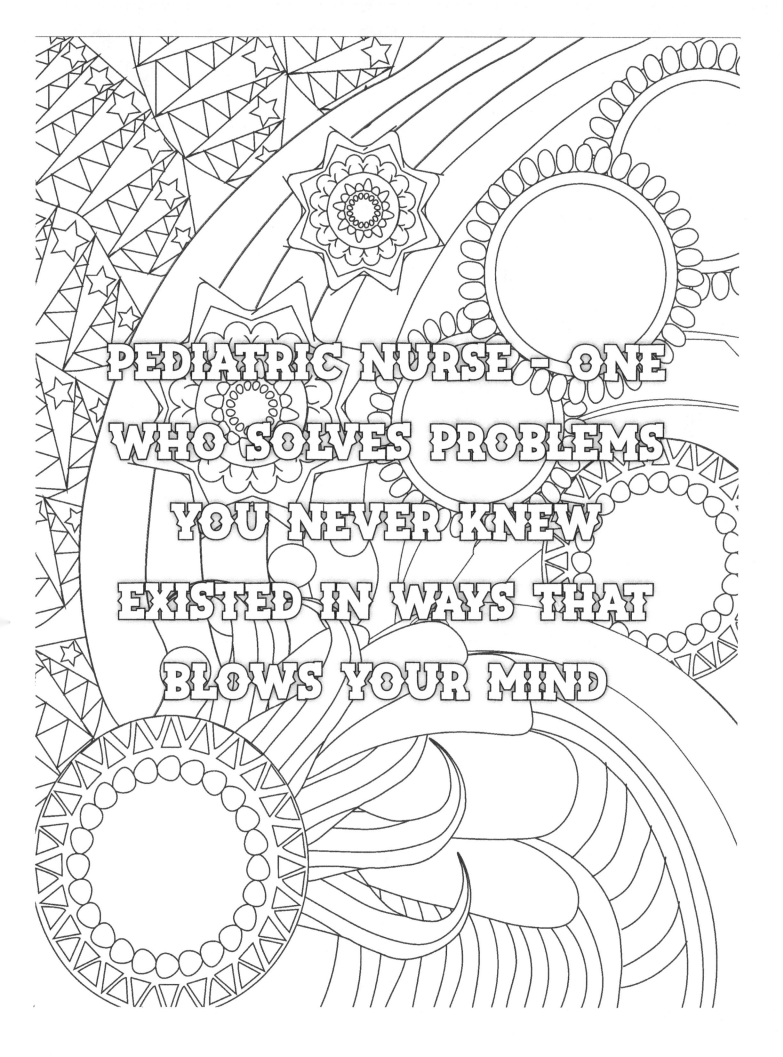

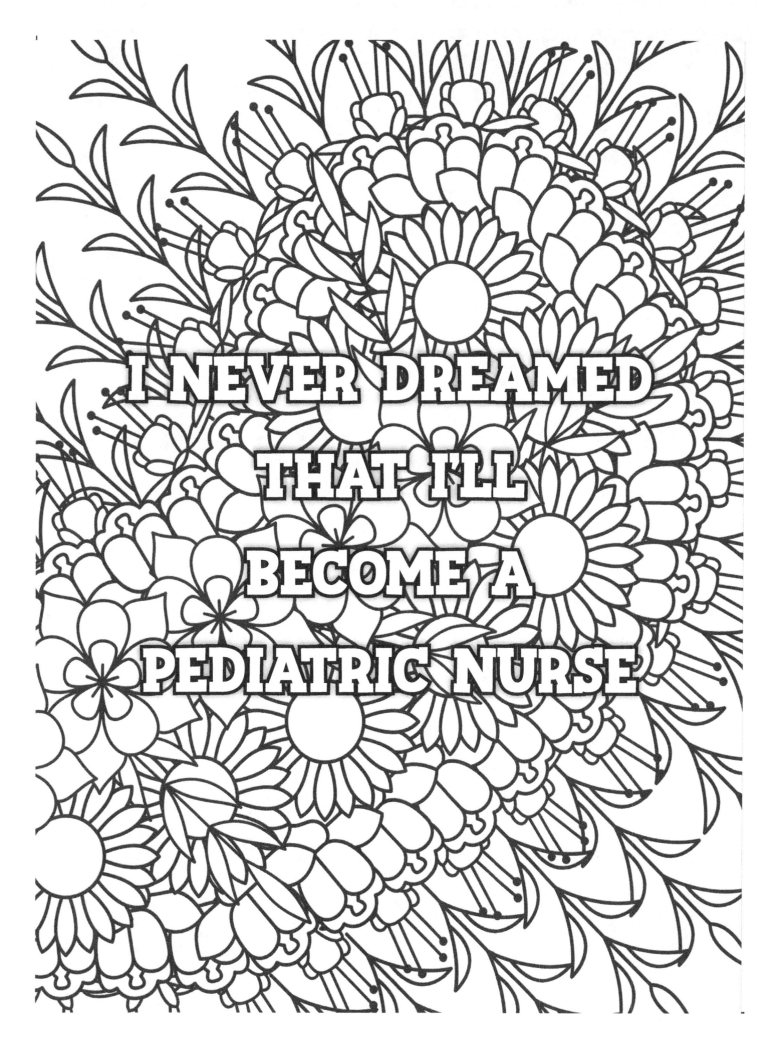

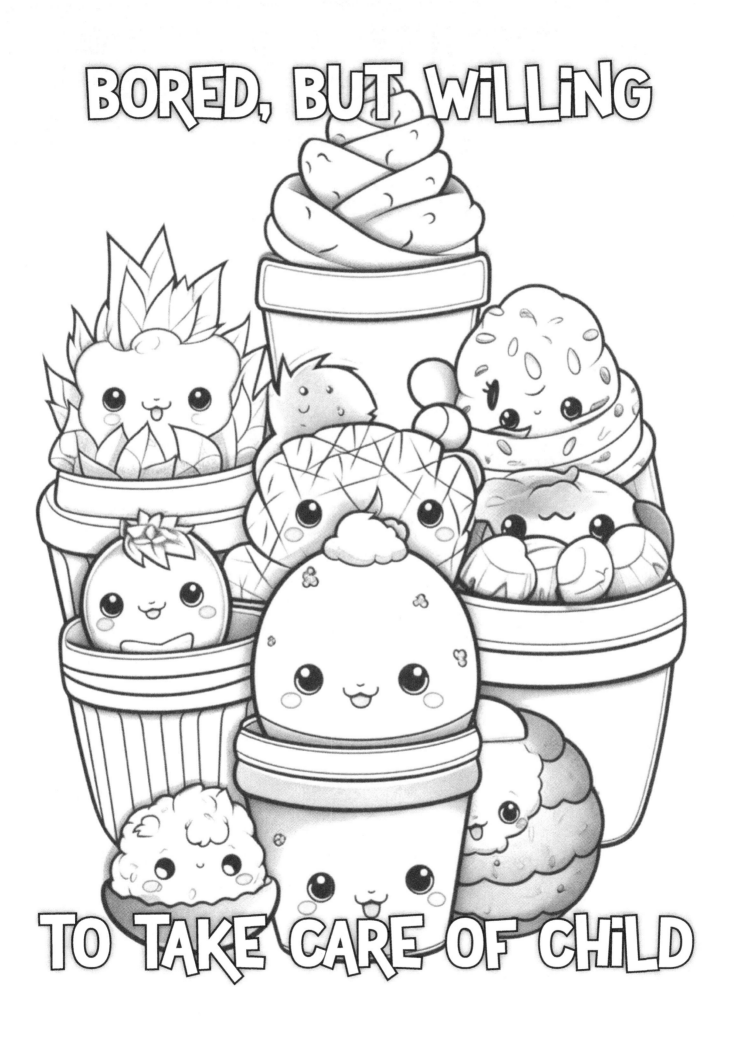

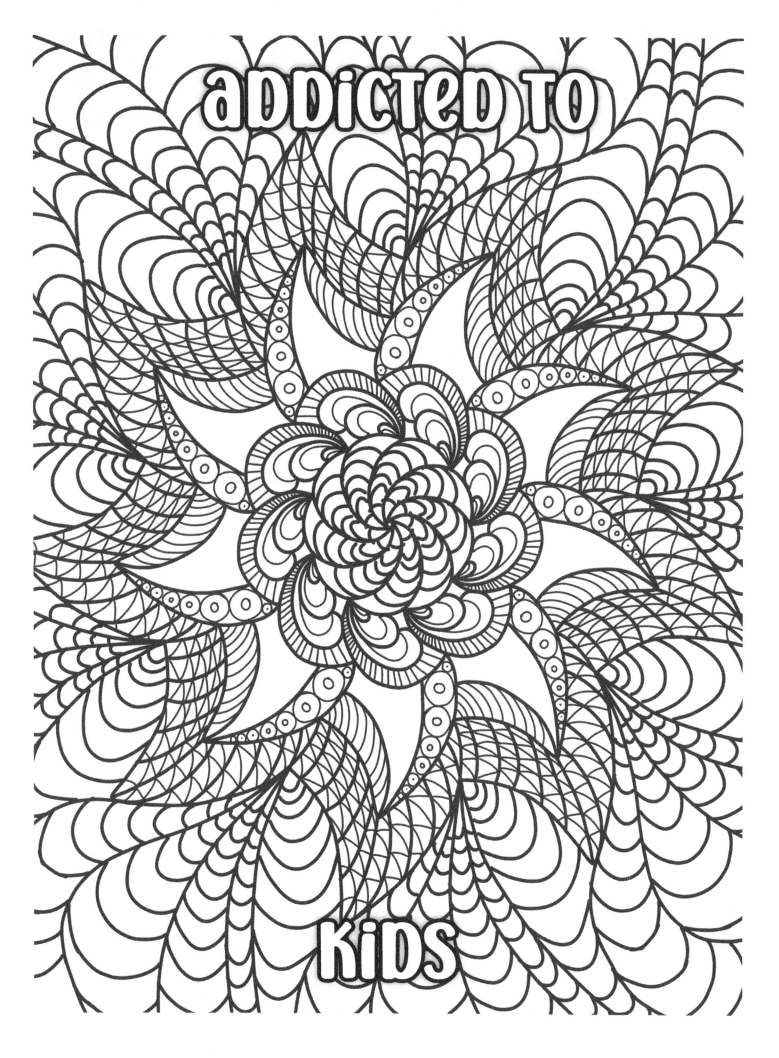

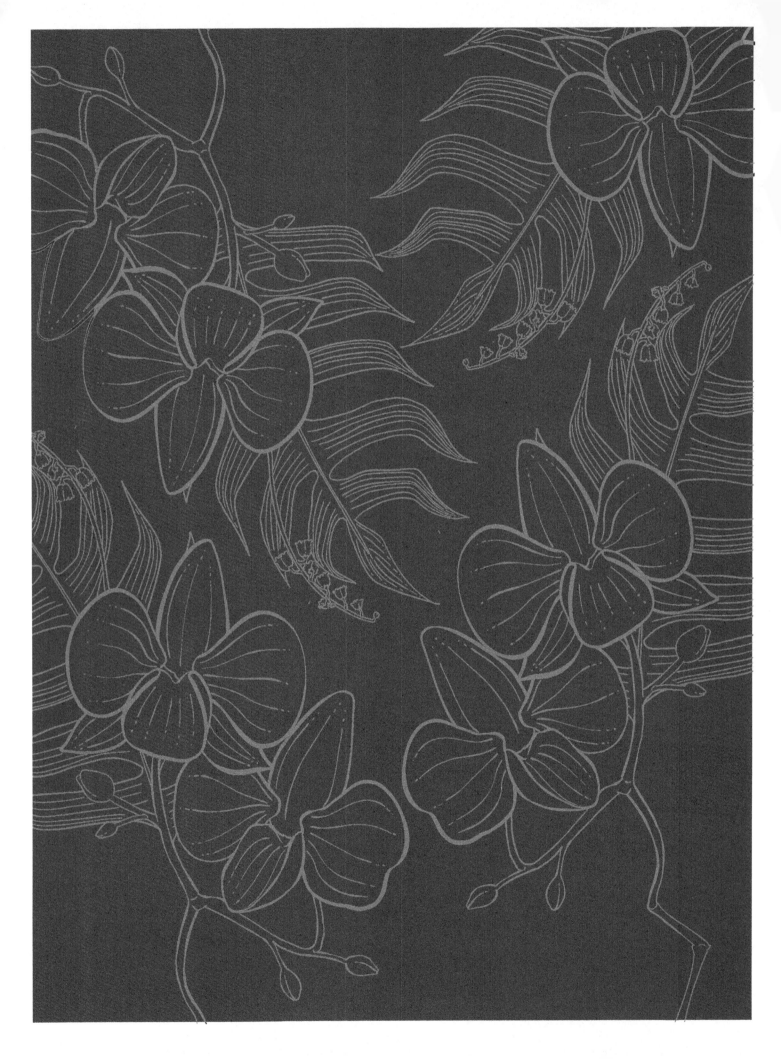

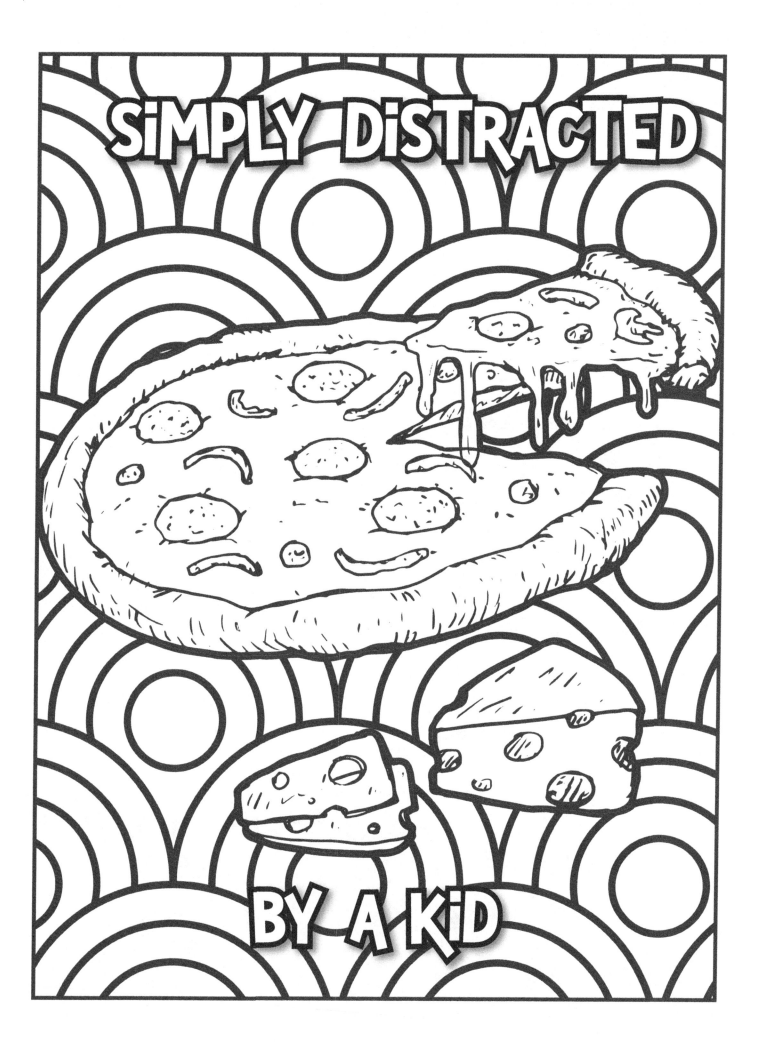

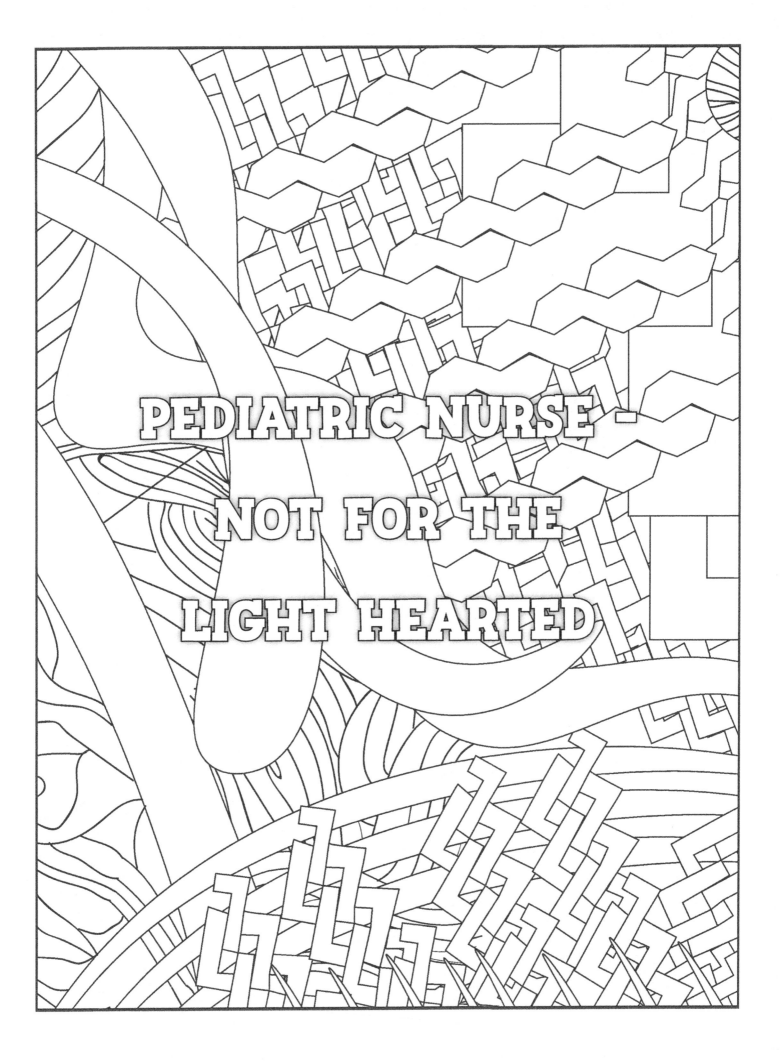

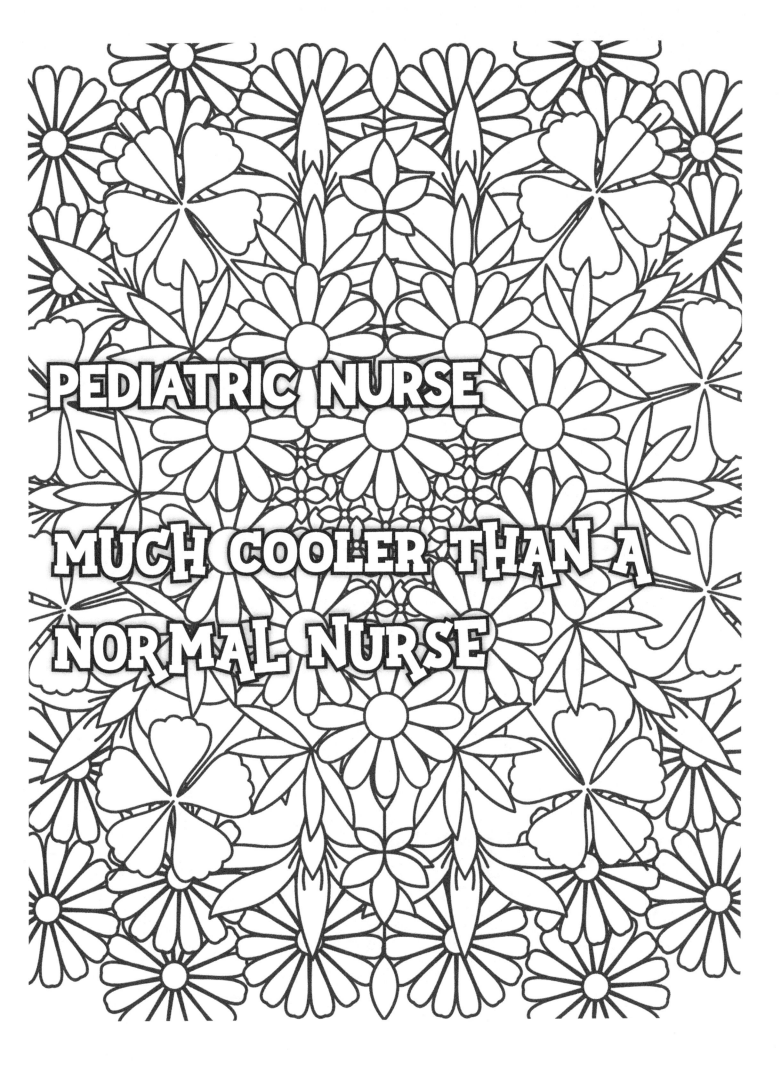

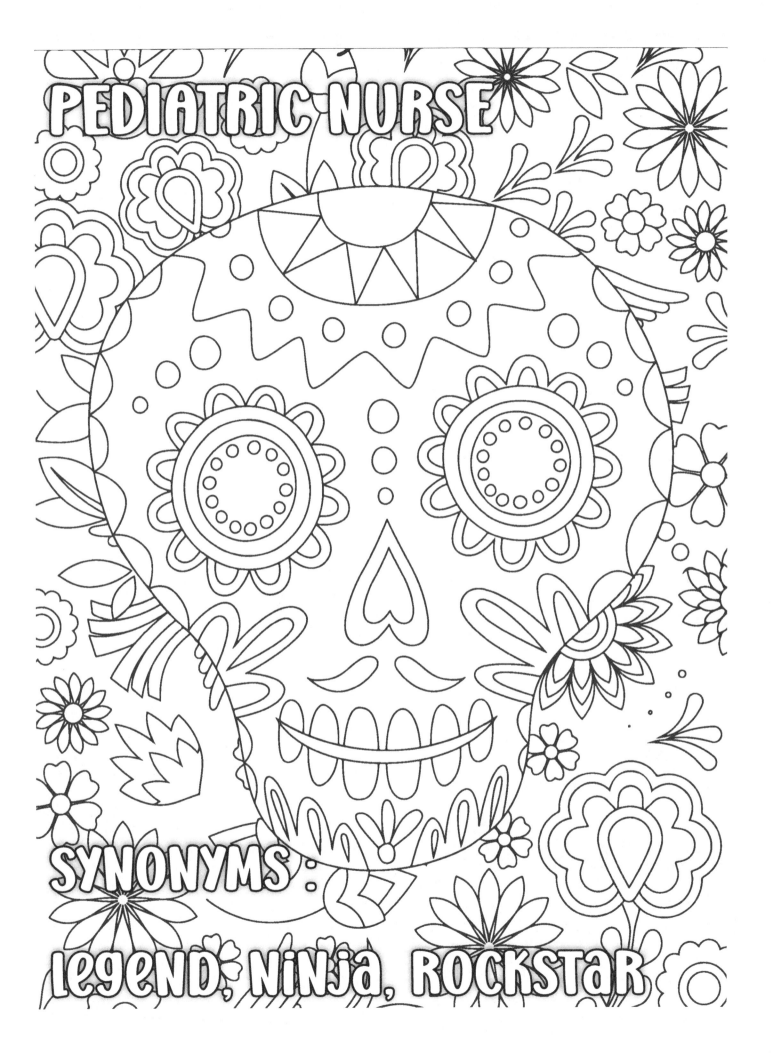

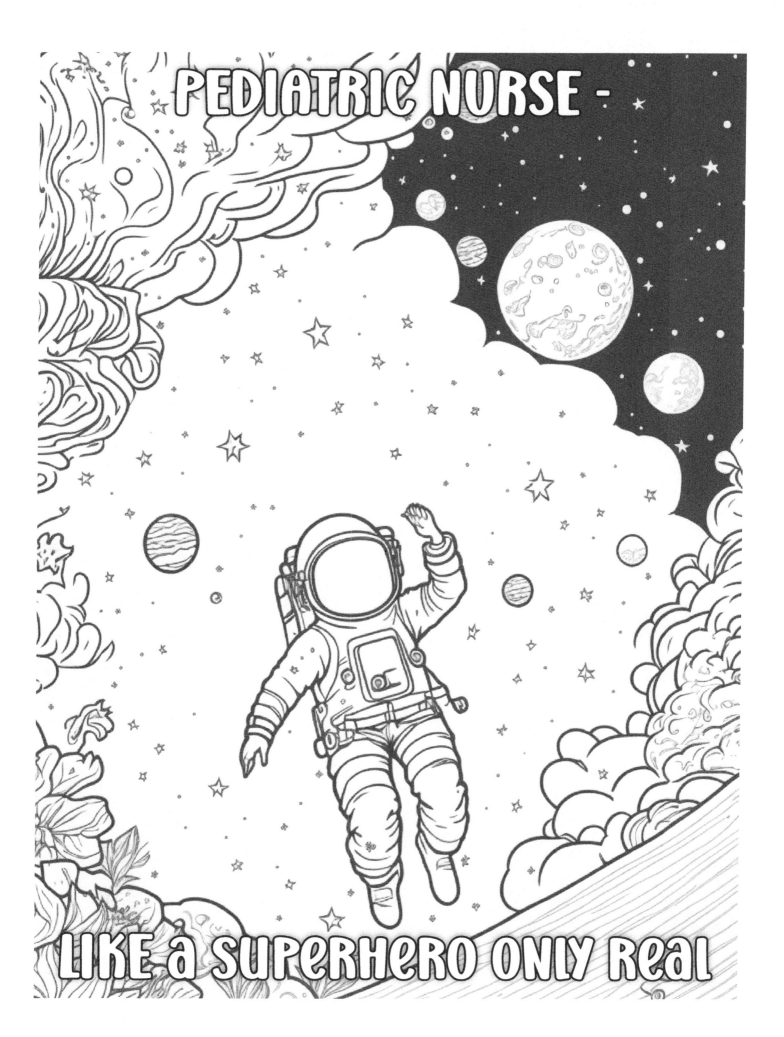

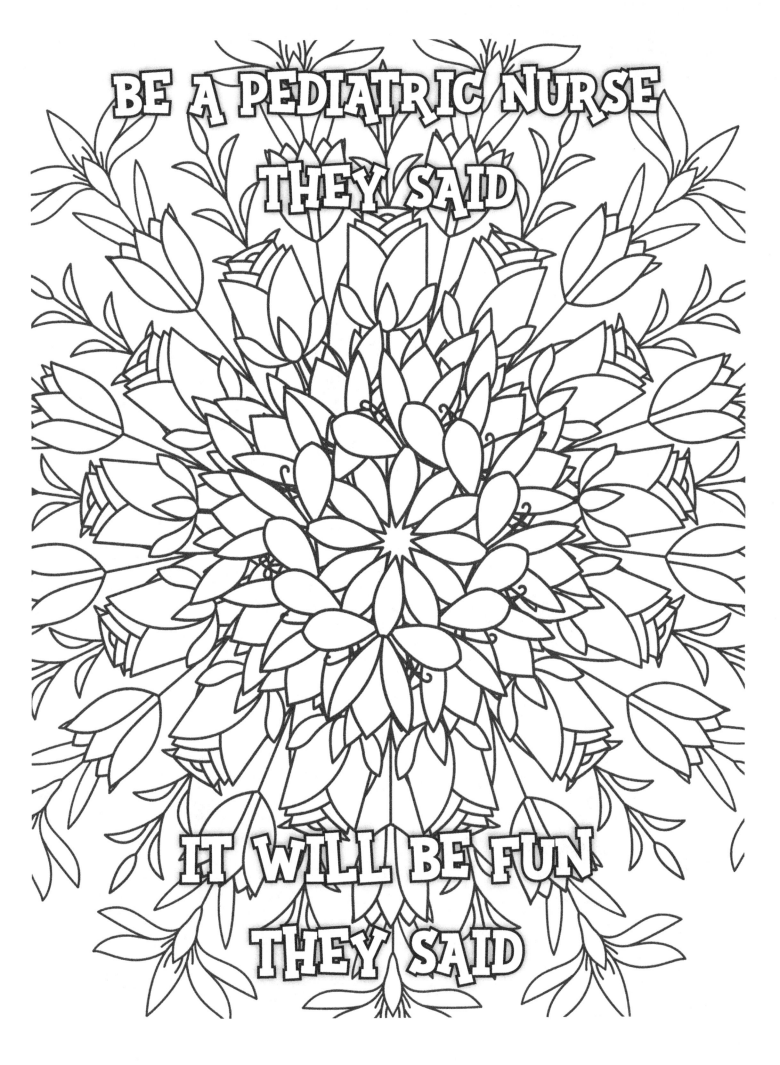

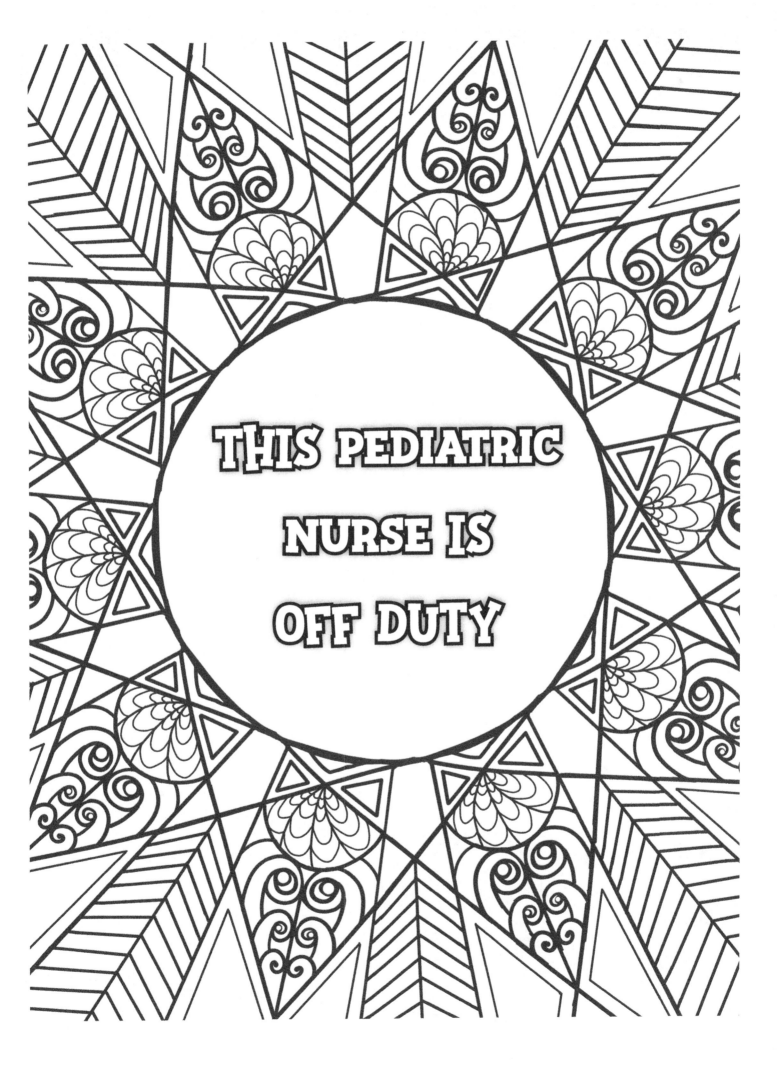

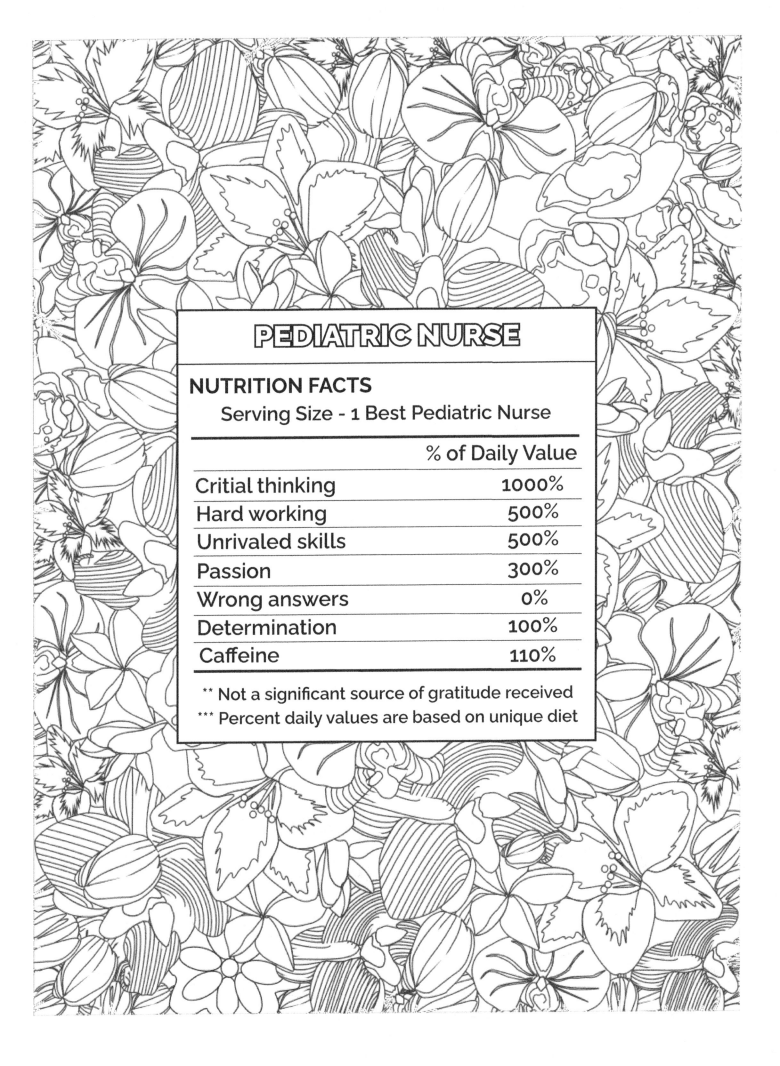

PEDIATRIC NURSE

NUTRITION FACTS

Serving Size - 1 Best Pediatric Nurse

	% of Daily Value
Critial thinking	1000%
Hard working	500%
Unrivaled skills	500%
Passion	300%
Wrong answers	0%
Determination	100%
Caffeine	110%

** Not a significant source of gratitude received

*** Percent daily values are based on unique diet

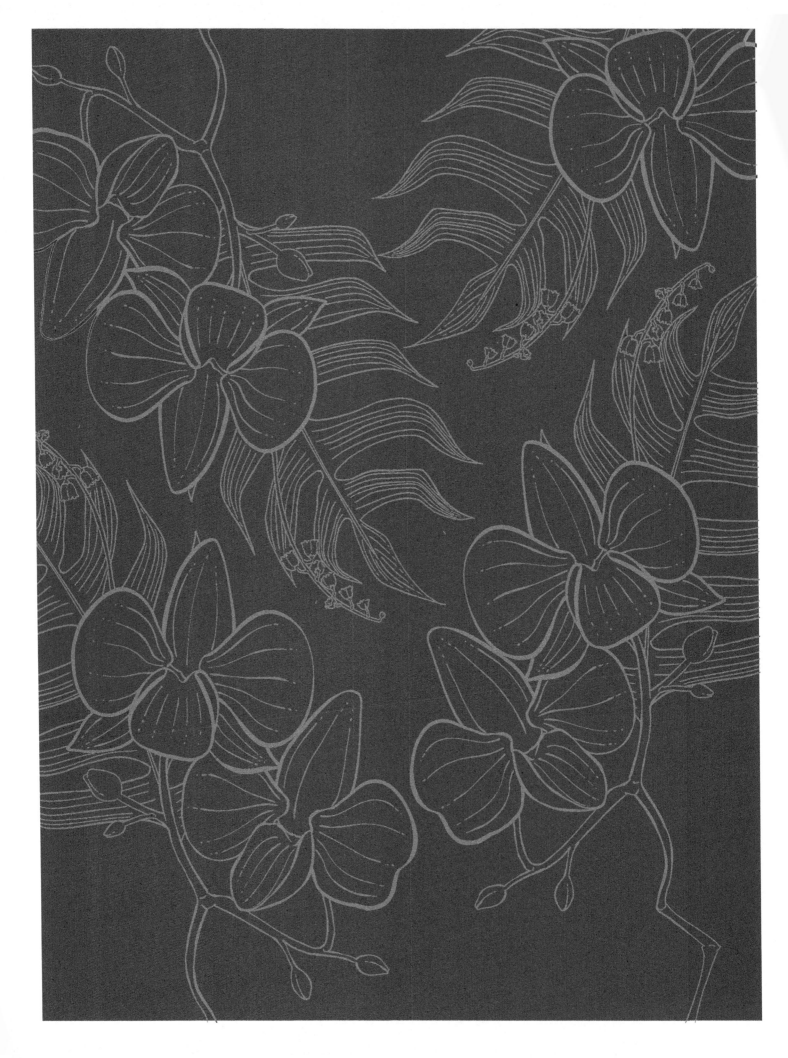